Activities for the Family Caregiver

ALZHEIMER'S DISEASE

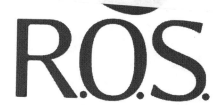

R.O.S.

HOW TO ENGAGE
HOW TO LIVE

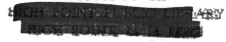
Scott Silknitter, Cindy Bradshaw,
Robert D. Brennan, Vanessa Emm,
Linda Redhead, Alisa Tagg, and Dawn Worsley

Disclaimer

This book is for informational purposes only and is not intended as medical advice, a diagnosis, or treatment. Always seek advice from a qualified physician about medical concerns, and do not disregard medical advice because of something you read in this book. This book does not replace the need for diagnostic evaluation, ongoing physician care, and professional assessment of treatments. Every effort has been made to make this book as complete and helpful as possible. It is important, however, for this book to be used as a resource and idea-generating guide and not as an ultimate source for a plan of care.

Published by
R.O.S. Therapy Systems, L.L.C.
Greensboro, NC
888-352-9788
www.ROSTherapySystems.com

Introduction:
Activities for the Family
Caregiver—Alzheimer's Disease

This book is a general guide to Activities for the Family Caregiver of someone with Alzheimer's disease. Designed for the family caregiver, this book was co-authored by multiple national experts with nearly 200 years of elder and dementia care experience.

This book is based on the principles and approaches used by the National Certification Council for Activity Professionals (NCCAP) and the National Association of Activity Professionals (NAAP) for the training and/or certification of long-term care and activity professionals. Since 1982 these organizations have been at the forefront of quality of life issues for seniors, their families, and their caregivers.

This book incorporates common sense and practical information for engaging your loved one who has Alzheimer's disease. Whether it is leisure activities or activities of daily living, our goal is for family caregivers to have this much-needed information at their fingertips whenever they need it.

It is my sincere hope that you find this book helpful. Our family knows and understands that feeling of, "What do we do?" I encourage you to have other family members and caregivers of your loved one read it as well. Doing so will enable everyone who is involved in caring for your loved one to be consistent with their approach, verbal cues, physical assistance, and modifications that can produce positive results.

From our family of caregivers to yours, please remember that you are not alone, and to never give up.

Scott Silknitter

Table of Contents

**Family Members and Caregivers
that have read this book:**

_____

_____

_____

_____

_____

_____

_____

_____

_____

_____

_____

_____

_____

Chapter 1

Alzheimer's Disease Overview and Symptoms

It is very emotional and frightening as you or your loved one begin to suspect the possibility of memory problems developing. You may feel overwhelmed, resentful, or angry. This is absolutely normal! It is important to know what is considered normal aging and what may be early symptoms of Alzheimer's disease.

It is **_essential_** when an individual is experiencing memory problems or confusion to undergo a thorough medical evaluation to rule out potential illnesses with symptoms which mimic dementia.

Most individuals over 65 will experience some type of forgetfulness. This is considered part of the normal aging process.

Dementia is not a specific disorder or disease, but a syndrome (group of symptoms) associated with a progressive loss of memory and other intellectual functions which seriously interfere with performing various tasks.

Beside Alzheimer's and other known diseases associated with dementia, these symptoms can be caused by nearly 40 other different diseases and conditions, ranging from dietary deficiencies and metabolic disorders, to head injuries and inherited diseases. These conditions can exhibit or mimic the symptoms of dementia and many are considered "Reversible Dementia" and are treatable.

The most common cause of dementia, Alzheimer's disease, usually progresses over an eight to ten-year period. The progression of Alzheimer's is as challenging for family caregivers as it is for their loved one.

With Alzheimer's, your loved one's cognitive ability slowly declines affecting parts of their brain causing issues with memory, language, judgment, mood and behaviors, spatial abilities, and motor skills.

Memory

An initial symptom of Alzheimer's disease is memory loss. Memory loss varies depending on the person and what "stage" their dementia might be in at that time. There might be moments of lucidity, when your loved one might remember specific details of people, places, and events. You must cherish those moments and learn to recognize them no matter what form they come in. The movie *The Notebook* displayed this well. The woman in the movie with dementia could not remember her children or their names, but she felt a familiar comfort with them. On occasion, she would also recognize her husband when he played "their" song. They would dance and discuss the children. Then suddenly, she would look up from dancing and not know who the man was in front of her or why they were dancing.

Dementia damages parts of the brain. The area of the brain that stores new memories is damaged first. That is why people with Alzheimer's live in the past, and all caregivers need to know the person your loved one was their whole life. Your loved one may be an 82-year-old living in their 32-year-old memories. You and all caregivers must accept this, and get to know that 32-year-old who shows up in your 82-year-old loved one on any given day.

In the early stages, people tend to forget little details of the day, such as appointments, or misplacing items they use daily, such as car keys, wallet, or reading glasses. Leaving themselves notes may help initially.

People also realize at this point that they are having memory issues and may try to cover it up. For example, you and your husband had been reviewing insurance policies and bills one weekend to prepare for an upcoming meeting with your agent. For 30 years, your husband was meticulous about files and putting things away properly so they were readily available when you needed them.

The day of the meeting, you realize the files you need are not in the cabinet. You ask your husband where they are and if he put them back after you reviewed them over the weekend. He may respond with, "I put them on the kitchen counter because we would need them later this week," which he would never have done before. The truth may be he simply couldn't remember where he had put them.

In the middle stages, people may start to forget more recent events, such as a phone call, or a visitor, or if they took their medicines. Often during this stage, the person tends to get a bit angry with their caregiver or loved ones. They know and insist they took their medicine, but they can't explain why the pills are still in the daily caddy. They say, "Someone must have refilled the dispenser." That one small issue can become very frustrating for them.

At the end stages, your loved one will recall very few recent or past events. At this stage, they may combine a past and present life event. They may start telling you what they ate for lunch and then share that their mother made the meal.

Language

Communication can be a significant challenge with dementia. For your loved one, it may be something as simple as not being able to find the "right" word to describe something or not finding the words to use at all. A great example of this is when you ask your loved one a question, she turns her head the other way and stares into space. This may seem as if she doesn't understand the question, but it may simply be her processing the information which is taking longer than what you are accustomed to.

Your loved one may also become repetitive in her speech. She focuses on one phrase or sentence and uses this phrase over and over again when answering questions.

Something to keep in mind when communicating is your body language and nonverbal actions. This can be a challenge in a heated or frustrated moment when one is having a "bad day," but studies have shown 90% of the communication involving individuals with Alzheimer's disease is nonverbal. Things like eye contact, body movements, gestures, and touching often take the place of verbal responses. We will address this further in Chapter 4, Communicating and Motivating for Success.

Judgment

Your loved one's judgment will be affected in several ways with dementia, from picking out clothes, to cooking, to making choices that put their physical or financial safety at risk.

Clothing and picking out what they will wear may be a sign that your loved one's judgment might be slipping a bit. Your loved one might begin:

- Meshing colors that they never would have before.

- Layering items, such as wearing three or four shirts on top of each other.

The layering of items may happen because they did not remember they had put the first shirt on before adding another.

One of the tips which we will discuss in detail later in this book is to have clothing "laid out" the night before they are worn. Another option is to pick out one week's worth of clothing combinations and place one outfit on a hanger for each day of the week. This not only saves time and frustration during dressing, but may save Mom unspoken embarrassment in public if she realizes her clothing does not match.

Beyond clothing, physical safety is a concern starting with what has been considered minor everyday tasks. For example, a person can become so immersed with an activity that they may let time slip away and be late to pick up a child from a school event that isn't routine. An individual with Alzheimer's may forget the child all together.

When looking at physical safety, a person with Alzheimer's may go out for a walk and not be able to find their way back.

Cooking is another serious issue that needs to be addressed. Your loved one with Alzheimer's may start cooking something on the stove and may walk away without remembering they started it. They may also try cooking something like a frozen pizza in a conventional oven by placing it on a plastic, microwave-safe plate that melts, ruins the oven, and possibly catches on fire.

Decreased judgment related to finances can also become a significant issue. It may start with something as simple as using a $50 bill to pay for a pizza instead of a $20 bill, but can grow into something that many people experience today. The person may have been worried about their money at an earlier stage of Alzheimer's. They may have hidden money in odd spots around their home, such as between their box spring and mattress, or in a refrigerator drawer. As their disease progresses, they may forget where they placed it at a time they need to pay for something like medication.

The decreased judgment associated with the progression of Alzheimer's can seem daunting in many ways, but can be overcome and worked through with proper planning and oversight.

Mood and Behaviors

Changes in mood or exhibiting behaviors that family members have never seen are often the most convincing evidence for families that something is wrong!

The moods or behaviors can come in many forms, such as being stubborn, resisting care, pacing, wandering, using obscene or abusive language, stealing, hiding things, engaging in inappropriate sexual behavior, urinating in unsuitable places, eating inappropriate objects, and dropping lit cigarettes.

Please remember that it is the disease causing these changes in your loved one. They did not choose to have Alzheimer's, but it has happened, and now they are saying and doing things that you never thought possible. We will address simple techniques to work with behavioral changes later in the book.

One other area that we need to touch on related to behaviors is sundowning. Sundowning refers to the increased confusion that many individuals with Alzheimer's disease experience during sunset hours. Many dementia individuals are friendly and calm, until about 3:00–4:30 in the afternoon. They start to become restless and may be seen as uncooperative. Many symptoms can be exhibited at this time. We can analyze and look for triggers, but it may not have anything to do with an event or an action that occurred. Remember, most of the time the issues have nothing to do with you, the caregiver, even though it may feel like a behavior or emotion is being directed at you.

It simply just "is."

No one knows for sure what brings on sundowning, but several potential causes/triggers have been attributed to this syndrome which include things, such as:

- Frequent napping during the day which leaves the individual awake in the evening.

- Change in the lighting or the warmth that comes during the day and goes away in the evenings.

Regardless of why, the issue of behaviors changing in the evening is real and often can be more frustrating to the caregiver than to the individual with the disease.

Remember this syndrome is caused by the disease, not by choice. This is easier said than done, but exercising patience and understanding may be the best way to begin combatting this behavior.

Spatial Abilities

Spatial abilities are those that allow a person to think or visualize items three-dimensionally and solve problems. For example, they are trying to walk in the house from a carpeted area to a tile area, and they think they have to step down or step up. Another example is that a black welcome mat could appear as a hole, and your loved one may try to step over it or walk around it.

Another example can be in a bathroom with a white toilet and solid white tile flooring. It may be difficult to judge the depth of the toilet seat between the floor and the seat when sitting.

Motor Skills

As your loved one's Alzheimer's disease progresses, it will begin to affect their motor skills as well. This will affect their ability to perform basic tasks, such as walking, dressing, and eating a meal.

No matter the cause, there are several general symptoms that your loved one may experience. As the primary caregiver, you must be as prepared and flexible as possible to handle them. On any given day, you may not know what kind of day you will have until your loved one is awake and the day has begun. If you notice that something is different and that they are starting on the path to a "bad day," look for any reason, no matter how small, that could be the trigger.

A trigger can cause a behavior in your loved one that is inappropriate. Something as simple as a commercial on television could trigger an emotion or frustration from when your loved one served in the war. Providing an opportunity for your loved one to reminisce and talk about the war in a positive way can be less stressful than stating the war is over. Gently bringing your loved one out of the trigger can be more beneficial for both of you than arguing.

Now that we have reviewed what some of the symptoms of your loved one's dementia might be, please note that many functions may remain intact and they will vary from individual to individual.

Alzheimer's can best be explained by the three-stage model:

Stage 1: Early/Mild
(lasts approximately 2–4 years)

- Frequent memory loss, especially with conversations and attending events.

- Problems with language, both receptive and expressive.

- Forgets where items are placed.

- Forgets where car is parked.
- Needs reminders for routine daily activities.

Stage 2: Middle/Moderate
(lasts approximately 2–10 years)

- Pervasive and persistent memory loss.
- Forgetfulness about personal history.
- Inability to recognize friends and family.
- May become lost.
- Sleep patterns may change.
- Assistance required with all "Activities of Daily Living" (ADLs)—bathing, dressing, toileting, transferring, and mobility.
- Behavior episodes—increased agitation, anger, and/or sundowning.
- Incontinence of bowel and bladder.
- Supervision and assistance with meals.
- Loss of mobility and coordination.

During this stage, there is a high risk of falls and other accidents. Coordination and balance are affected as well as attention span.

Stage 3: Late/Severe
(lasts approximately 1–3 years)

- Loss of ability to communicate.
- Nutrition becomes a problem due to swallowing problems.
- Unable to process information.
- Severe to total loss of verbal skills.
- Will require total care for all activities of daily living.
- Cannot walk, usually bedridden.

Now that we have touched on the general symptoms that your loved one may experience, the following chapters discuss the benefits, "How To's," preparation, and execution of activities for your loved one.

We use an approach based on decades of experience and proven strategies which can be accomplished by using the techniques based on the Four Pillars of Activities.

Chapter 2

Activities, Their Benefits, and the Family

Activities are anything and everything. It can be a conversation, folding towels, taking a walk, playing a game, getting dressed, or watching a movie. The key for all family caregivers is learning the simple techniques that work for their loved one which allow for success.

Familiarity with people, activities, and routine is so important to our loved ones. To understand this better, think about your own life. We are creatures of habit, are we not? When we attend church, we sit in the same pew. When we go out to eat Chinese food, we go to the same restaurant. When we talk to people, we are most comfortable talking to people with whom we have something in common. Routine becomes a part of us at a very early age. As your loved one begins to lose their memories of current/recent events, they start to cling to their memories from the past. The urgency of routine, consistency, activities, family, and friends becomes even more relevant.

New things can and should be tried, but having consistency is good with this disease.

As we focus on the familiar for our loved one, we must also prepare ourselves, other family members, and friends that Mom may look and sound the same on the outside, but because of her dementia, she is not the same person we remember from the past.

Visits from family and friends should be welcomed and encouraged, but prior to the visit, some preparation will be needed to allow the visit to be successful and as stress free as possible.

**Consistency** is key! Provide visitors with a schedule of events with regard to the daily items, such as mealtimes, grooming activities, and favorite routines.

Another thing that might minimize the stress during a family visit and after, is for you to prepare the visitor for the types of things they might see. You are the primary family caregiver, and you are the one who must deal with any issues that arise long after visitors or temporary caregivers have gone home. Visits from family and friends are important. Please prepare everyone as much as possible prior to the visit so any inadvertent triggers of bad behavior or other issues can be minimized.

The Benefits of Activities with a Standard Approach

Caregiver Benefits

As a caregiver, how many times have you wished to sit and enjoy just three minutes of peace, or be able to sit and drink a cup of coffee while it is still warm, or have one daily routine run smoothly? Planned and well-executed activities can result in less stress for you and your loved one and may just give you that little bit of time. Whether the activity involves playing a game or bathing, pre-planning as many details as possible can make a significant, positive difference for everyone.

When your loved one is actively engaged and participating in a reminiscing-type activity, such as looking at pictures in photo albums, it allows your loved one the opportunity to feel relaxed. This in return gives you, the caregiver, the same opportunity to feel relaxed. It also provides an opportunity to converse and reminisce about past experiences.

Social Benefits of Activities

Engaging your loved one in a variety of activities can have the same positive effects that they experienced through positive social interactions throughout their entire lives. Whether it is between you and your loved one, or your loved one and someone else, the positive social benefits can come in a variety of forms, including intellectual, emotional, spiritual, and physical.

Intellectual: Participating in social activities like board games or word games can help to support areas in the brain that can stimulate cognition and help prevent decline involved with age-related dementia. Any type of activity that allows an individual to think/ponder a response, can be beneficial to both the caregiver and their loved one allowing for a more meaningful interaction.

Emotional: It just makes us "feel good" to have a pleasant interaction with another human being. Think about your life and all of the evenings out with friends you have had over the years, when you were having so much fun that you did not want the night to end. Just because someone has Alzheimer's does not mean that their reaction to positive interaction will be any different. In fact, positive interactions with others can be very important in reducing stress and reducing psychological problems, such as depression and anxiety.

Those interactions that may start with one activity can lead to others. For example, looking at a photo album may prompt a discussion about a family reunion, which could lead to a discussion about a wedding, and then a discussion about a song that was playing at your loved one's wedding. Little things matter. You never know where an activity or a conversation can take you.

__Spiritual:__ Socialization in activities helps to ensure that one's belief system remains fluid throughout the transitions of living. Bible studies, prayer groups, prayers, and other services that support the need to connect and fellowship can be very beneficial. These activities help maintain and even strengthen faith and hope, and provide an understanding of existence.

__Physical:__ The old adage of "use it or lose it" comes into play with regard to the physical functioning of individuals. The more we exercise and do physical types of activities, the better it is for our overall health and well-being. Participating in physical activities together, such as walking or stretching, can help promote an increased functional ability. Physical activity causes a release of endorphins, which are "feel good happy feelings" that our bodies create naturally.

<u>Behavioral Benefits of Activities</u>

Well-planned and well-executed activities of any type can reduce challenging behaviors that sometimes arise when caring for someone with dementia.

Behaviors are nothing more than a means of communication when words are no longer effective. Keeping this in mind allows for you, the caregiver, to find understanding when a behavior occurs. Activity opportunities that can assist when challenging behavior occurs are in the form of redirection, such as going for a walk, moving into another room in the house, or focusing on what is on the walls, like pictures.

Distraction can be most helpful. Caregivers can often control difficult situations by distracting their loved one and/or avoiding those events or items that could lead to problems.

For example, if a person gets agitated by the sound of the garbage truck collecting trash once per week because it is a faint, but disruptive noise, perhaps that day would be a good day for a favorite activity, such as baking cookies. Trash pickup day could then become a "good day" for your loved one and ward off a potentially negative behavior.

Knowing a person's strengths and weaknesses will also assist in meaningful activity and behavioral changes. Concentrate on the activities they can do and the most appropriate times for them to do those activities. If they are more energetic in the morning, then the physical activities would be most beneficial then. If they are more agitated in the afternoon, that's when the less strenuous, more relaxing types of activities, such as listening to or playing favorite music, or being read to might be more appropriate.

Know your own strengths and weaknesses as well. When do you need a break? What do you enjoy doing?

If you know that the caregiver coming later in the day has a special interest in reading the Bible, then leave that for them to do with your loved one.

<u>Self-Esteem Benefits of Activities</u>

Leisure activities offered at the right skill level provide your loved one with an opportunity for success. Any time we can do something for ourselves we feel better than having someone else do that task for us. Think about a time when you were working on a project and the sense of satisfaction you had when you finished it. That feeling is the same for everyone—no matter what the task or activity is.

Small or large, from brushing teeth to creating original art pieces, each of us enjoys the satisfaction and praise from accomplishing something. The more opportunities we give someone to participate in and accomplish something, the more they will feel empowered and willing to participate in other activities.

When engaging your loved one, your goal will always be to enhance their self-worth and self-esteem. We must remember that your ability to be flexible and go with the flow is an important part of that process as well when working with someone who has Alzheimer's.

Here is an example of what we mean. Billy loved to play Pinochle. As his Alzheimer's progressed, he forgot the rules and would often make up new rules to the game. The family had two choices. They could spend their time correcting Billy each time he did something wrong, or they could go with the flow and just enjoy playing and watching the look on his face when he won every game.

Sleep Benefits of Activities

Alzheimer's disease and sundowning can play havoc with an individual's sleep patterns. Engagement and activities can have a direct benefit to sleep patterns for everyone. The more active a person is during the day, the more likely the person may be to sleep better throughout the night.

While the person may sleep/nap during the day, if you keep a set schedule, dim the lights around the nap times, and bring the person closer to the light during awake times, they will adapt to their surroundings.

When waking, the sooner you get your loved one to brighter lights the better. At bedtime, the more dim the room the better. This sets the mood or the tone of the event.

Schedule many activities of interest throughout the day to keep the person as awake as possible during the day—tire them out if you will.

Keep sleep and awake schedules as routine as possible.

Family and Other Caregivers

"Leisure Activities" and "Activities of Daily Living" are critical aspects to caring for a loved one at home. Both types, leisure and daily living, require knowledge of your loved one's habits, preferences, abilities, and routines. This knowledge will enhance the ability of all caregivers to communicate and execute a planned activity with your loved one. Life happens, and things can happen spontaneously, but all activities should be planned to offer the best possible outcome to enhance your loved one's sense of well-being and to promote or enhance their physical, cognitive, and emotional health. In this book, we will focus on leisure activities and the activities of daily living with common sense suggestions and tips on the "How To's" of getting your loved one engaged, dressed, and fed.

This book was made for the millions of families and informal caregivers who care for their loved ones with some form of dementia at home. Recognizing the growth in the numbers of those aging in place due to financial need or desire to just be at home, the R.O.S. Activities 101/201 Programs and this book are based on the principles and approaches used by the professionals in skilled settings. This was done for two reasons.

1. Provide family caregivers the basic knowledge and tools to allow them to engage their loved one so that both can enjoy the benefits of activities.

2. Offer a starting point that will provide continuity of approach regarding care,

communication, and information-gathering to minimize changes and acclimation time if your loved one does have to move from home to an institutional setting.

If you choose to use the services of a home care agency while caring for your loved one at home, please ask if they have a Home Care Certified professional on staff, and make sure that the caregiver you choose has received basic training on Leisure Activities and Activities of Daily Living. This will assist with continuity of approach, communication, and planning that will benefit both you and your loved one.

Our goal is to improve your quality of life and the quality of life for the one you care for. We want to help you deliver meaningful programs of interest to your loved one that focus on physical, social, spiritual, cognitive, and recreational activities. Everyone involved in the care for your loved one should be "on the same page" to minimize changes and challenges that your loved one will face.

For someone who has Alzheimer's, consistent routine or continuity of approach provides that person a feeling of comfort and security. They are slowly losing their physical, cognitive, and social abilities. We owe it to our loved ones to make it a priority to preserve the independence they currently possess for as long as possible. We must remember that as the disease progresses, even the smallest things, like where you place the fork next to the plate, or how you respond to a loved one's question, could either elicit a positive interaction or create an atmosphere where your loved one feels lost, insecure, and worthless.

Not all family members may understand or accept your loved one's dementia or disease. Your loved one may look the same on the outside and might be having a "good day" when someone comes to visit. Family members who visit occasionally may not understand or see all of the symptoms that primary caregivers see daily. They may underestimate or minimize the responsibilities or stress. This can create conflict.

We recently worked with a family that was caring for their father at home. Most of the family members—his wife, two adult daughters, and their husbands—understood where Dad was in the disease. The son, however, had a hard time accepting Dad's Alzheimer's and its progression.

His daughters and his wife were involved every day in Dad's care and routines. The son came to visit every other week or so and would walk into the house with his typical greeting of, "Hey Dad." Dad would usually respond with, "Hey Bud, how's work? How's the family?" That gave a false sense of security to the son, who felt that Dad perhaps wasn't as bad as his sister stated. While he was in denial, he would say and do things that upset the normal routine that Mom and his sisters had settled into and adjusted for Dad as the disease progressed.

The son was in denial, and it took an outside professional to challenge the son with exercises that would engage his father in a higher level of conversation. The professional had the son do some brain aerobics with Dad.

They started a fun game of name the family member. They used pictures of family members from 20 years earlier and pictures of them today. This is a powerful exercise. When the son showed pictures of family members from 20 years earlier, his father was able to identify every family member, but as the son started showing pictures of the same family members from the past six months, Dad was unable to identify the family members, even pictures of the son himself. This was a real eye-opener for the son, who now had to come to terms with what was happening with Dad and that he would need to change what he did in order to help the rest of the family.

If it helps to avoid a conflict or stress, please have family members read this book prior to a visit so they can begin to understand the monumental task that you face as a caregiver. Use visits and interactions as teaching moments.

It can take a while to learn new roles and responsibilities. It is critical, however, to have as many family members and friends involved in your loved one's life as possible. This is not just to show your loved one they are cared for and loved, but also to give you, the primary family caregiver, the occasional and much-needed break.

A common approach is key. Demand it!

The Four Pillars of Activities

The R.O.S. Activities 101/201 Programs focus on the Four Pillars of Activities. These are areas that all caregivers for your loved one should be familiar with to provide continuity of care and give your loved one the greatest opportunity for success to engage and improve the quality of life for everyone.

First Pillar of Activities: Know your Loved One—Information Gathering and Assessment

Have a Personal History Form completed. Know them—who they are, who they were, and what their functional abilities are today. Make sure all caregivers know this as well.

Second Pillar of Activities: Communicating and Motivating for Success

Communication is key. Each caregiver must know how to effectively communicate with your loved one and be consistent with techniques.

Third Pillar of Activities: Customary Routines and Preferences

As best as possible, maintain a routine and daily plan based on your loved one's needs and preferences.

Fourth Pillar of Activities: Planning and Executing Activities

Based on all of the information you have gathered about your loved one, you have the opportunity to offer engaging activities that are appropriate and meet your loved one's personal preferences.

Chapter 3

First Pillar of Activities:
Know Your Loved One— Information Gathering and Assessment

It is important, before you begin providing personal care, that you first recognize various personal attributes and abilities of your loved one and yourself. The more you know about your loved one's lifestyle, likes, and dislikes, the easier providing for their personal and leisure needs will be.

Alzheimer's may not affect your loved one's personality, but it does affect their ability to interpret and deal with their surroundings as they did in the past.

It is important to concentrate on what your loved one **_CAN DO_**, not on what they **_CAN NOT DO_**. The more you know about your loved one, the more effective you can be as a caregiver. Caregiving routines should be kept structured and regular.

For instance, Dee, a 76-year-old, enjoyed sleeping in late. She never considered herself to be a morning person and would be in a foul mood if she was awakened too early. Her day would start at about 10:00 a.m. as she would slowly get herself out of bed. Dee welcomed a cup of hot coffee with only cream and her daily newspaper. When she was done, she would shower, brush her teeth, and get dressed. Only then was she ready to face the world and truly start her day. Her morning routine was a quiet time for her. This is an important piece of information about Dee that all caregivers should know so the day starts off on a good note.

Dementia is a physical illness, not a mental illness. However, individuals may suffer from both. Phil had bouts of depression. Though he usually had a good sense of humor and enjoyed working a puzzle every day after lunch, there were times that his caregiver could not get Phil engaged. These were the days that Phil would stay in bed. He would stop eating, even if he was offered his favorite foods, and would easily become tearful. These were the times that his caregiver would just sit by his bedside and hold his hand to reassure him that he was not alone and that he was cared about.

Knowing your loved one is the First Pillar of Activities. Knowing their individual needs, interests, functional abilities, and capacities will assist you in knowing how to communicate with them and plan or engage in activities with them.

You and your loved one may have been very private people. Having Alzheimer's will change that. Gathering information and sharing with other caregivers is critical as your loved one's past pleasures, likes, and activities will become cornerstones of the communication process for everyone.

If there is something that happened years ago that you consider embarrassing or private, and you choose not to share the information, please note that one way or another, it will come out.

Whatever it was that you think is difficult to share, caregivers and family members that offer assistance are not there to judge you or your loved one on something that happened years or even decades ago. They are there to help you in your moment of need today. Knowing your loved one is vital to the communication process and allows all caregivers the opportunity to turn a "bad day" into a "good day" through proper communication techniques.

As the primary caregiver, you may already know most of the answers, but this is a good and necessary exercise for you, other family members, and other caregivers to execute. We suggest everyone fill out the R.O.S. Personal History Form which comes later in this book. As a starting point, you, the primary caregiver, are most likely able to provide the following basic information:

Basic Information

Name, preferred name to be called, age, and date of birth

Background Information

Place of birth, cultural/ethnic background, marital status, children (how many, and their names), religion/church, military service/employment, education level, and primary language spoken

Medical and Dietary/Nutritional Information

Any formal diagnosis, allergies, and food regimen/diets

Habits

Drinking/alcohol, smoking, exercise, and other things that are a daily habit

Physical Status

Abilities/limitations, visual aids, hearing deficits, speech, communication, hand dominance, and mobility/gait

Mental Status

Alertness, cognitive abilities/limitations, orientation to family, time, place, person, routine, etc.

Social Status

One-on-one interaction, being visited, communicating with others through written word or phone calls, other means

Emotional Status

Level of contentment, outgoing/withdrawn, extroverted/introverted, dependent/independent

Leisure Status

Past, present, and possible future interest

Vision Status

Any impairment they may have

Informal Assessments

Informal assessments are done through interviews, observation, and information gathered through other means. These will allow you and others to "fill in the blanks" of the R.O.S. Personal History Form.

Interviews

Interviews are conducted with your loved one, or with family members, friends, or significant others.

Observation

An observation is what you and others have seen or heard concerning your loved one, e.g., how they interact with others, their behavior, and their responses to questions or statements made by others. This includes body language and expressions. You have probably seen these interactions a thousand times and made a mental note whenever something stuck out. Now, you must write them down for your future use and for others.

Information Gathered Through Other Means

Make a request of family members or friends to help complete the Personal History Form at the back of this book. You also may download a copy of the Personal History Form at www.StartSomeJoy.com. Gather as much information as possible and share it with all caregivers—family, informal, and formal.

Your ability to identify past preferences is vital to the planning and execution of an activity, which we will cover in this book. Details matter. Let's look at a couple of examples— reading and watching television.

Four people might all say they like "watching TV," yet they might not actually have the same activity in mind.

- Person 1—Enjoys watching the news channels but not much else.

- Person 2—Enjoys afternoon soap operas but not evening television.

- Person 3—Enjoys watching game shows.

- Person 4—Enjoys watching movies and History channel programs.

Four people might all say they like "reading," yet they might not actually have the same activity in mind.

- Person 1—Enjoys reading the newspaper every morning.

- Person 2—Enjoys reading magazines and looking at the pictures.

- Person 3—Enjoys reading paperback novels, especially love stories.

- Person 4—Enjoys reading the Bible.

As you can see from these examples, details matter. Gather as much information as you can for yourself and all caregivers who may help with your loved one.

Functional Levels

In addition to the Personal History Form, you also need to look at your loved one's functional level. When planning meaningful activities based on individual interests, you need to also consider your loved one's functional abilities. You need to set them up for success based on what they are able to accomplish. There are several definitions of functional levels. For the purpose of this topic, we will address the following four functioning levels:

Level 1

Your loved one has good social skills. They are able to communicate. They are alert and oriented to person, place, and time, and they have a long attention span.

Level 2

Your loved one has less social skills and their verbal skills may also be impaired. Your loved one may have some behavior symptoms. They may need something to do, and may have an increased energy level, but they have a shorter attention span.

Level 3

Your loved one has less social skills. Their verbal skills are even more impaired than they were at Level 2. They are also easily distracted. Your loved one may have some visual/spatial perception and balance concerns, and they need maximum assistance with their care.

Level 4

Your loved one has a low energy level, nonverbal communication skills, and they rarely initiate contact with others, however, they may respond if given time and cues. With the personal history and functional level information, you and every caregiver have the greatest opportunity to provide person-appropriate activities for your loved one.

Chapter 4

Second Pillar of Activities:
Communicating and Motivating for Success

Communicating and motivating for success is the Second Pillar of Activities. The key to good communication is to be a good listener. This means listening with your ears and eyes. **_All_** caregivers must listen to the words that someone is speaking, as well as listen with their eyes to how their loved one is acting. Listening behavior can either enhance and encourage communication or shut down communication altogether. You need to assess your listening style and be able to assess the listening styles of the other caregivers and family members working with your loved one.

Verbal Communication

Communication is an interactive process where information is exchanged. The ability to respond appropriately and give feedback are important skills each caregiver must possess or learn.

Verbal Approaches

- Use exact, short, positive phrases. Repeat twice if necessary.

- Speak slowly with words they know.

- Give time for the person to answer.

- Give one instruction at a time.

- Use a warm, gentle tone of voice.

- There is no need to shout, unless the individual also has a hearing impairment.

- If the person is unable to see you because of a visual impairment, be sure to use verbal cues to let them know you are engaged.

- Talk to them like an adult.

Verbal Communication Tips

- Make your presence known when entering a room by saying hello and calling them by their name.

- Identify yourself. Do not assume your loved one knows who you are.

- If there are others present, address the person by name so there is no confusion as to whom you are talking.

- Indicate the end of a conversation, and let your loved one know when you leave.

- Speak directly to your loved one.

- Always answer questions, and be specific in your responses.

- When giving directions, make them as simple and clear as possible.

- When speaking with other caregivers about your loved one while they are present, make sure the conversation is respectful of your loved one. They may move or speak slowly, but assume that they hear everything.

Nonverbal Communication

Although it may seem that most communication happens with words, research has shown that actually most communication occurs through an individual's nonverbal actions and body language. There are five key elements to consider:

Facial Expressions

Be aware of what your facial expressions are conveying to your loved one. Your mood will be mirrored.

Eye Contact

Ensure that you have made eye contact with your loved one and that their attention is focused on you and what you are saying.

Gestures and Touch

Calmly use nonverbal signs, such as pointing, waving, and other hand gestures in combination with your words.

Tone of Voice

The inflection in your voice helps your loved one relate to the words you are saying.

Body Language

Be aware of the position of your hands and arms when talking to your loved one.

***Note:** When communicating with your loved one, be mindful that their body language may not fully tell how they feel or what they are trying to express because of slow movement. Your body language, however, will be read by your loved one.

Nonverbal Communication Tips

- Always approach your loved one from the front before speaking to them.
- Smile and extend your hand as to shake their hand. Use touch where welcomed.
- Be at eye level with the person you are talking to.

- Use nonverbal gestures along with words.

- Give nonverbal praises, such as smiles and head nods.

- Be an active listener.

- Make sure that all caregivers give your loved one the opportunity and time to speak.

Being a Detective

As your loved one's Alzheimer's progresses, there will be many days that you will not know what kind of day it will be until after the day has started.

Let us look at Millie and Pam. Pam had been hired by Millie's family as a five-day-per-week caregiver for Millie. For five years, Pam helped care for Millie and became part of the family. Pam knew she had a great relationship with Millie and had learned to communicate with her very well. Pam noticed that recently

Millie was becoming very aggressive in the afternoon and would attempt to leave the house.

This behavior can be scary for a family member and all caregivers. With dementia and behaviors like this, you must try to figure out each day where your loved one believes they are, how old they think they are, and what is happening. This means one day your loved one could be looking for their mom which indicates they believe they are very young. On another day they could be looking for their baby which would indicate they are now in their early 20's.

Once you can identify where your loved one is, you can then project what activities would be vital to them during that time period.

For Pam, she ran through the past few days in her mind looking for the smallest details or hints as to why Millie was so eager to get out of the house in the afternoon.

Then it dawned on her that over the past two days Millie made isolated comments like, "That girl better mind me and be right home."

Knowing that Millie had a daughter and that the behavior was occurring the same time each day, Pam thought Millie may be looking for her daughter to come home from school.

When Millie does not see her daughter, she begins to panic. Pam discussed the situation with the family, and they decided that each day one hour before the repeated incidents Pam would engage Millie in conversations about her daughter and about being a mother. Pam discovered that those conversations alone met the need of her client regarding her daughter. Sometimes it's not a quick answer. Sometimes it takes the caregiver and the families working together and trying various things. Even if you try something and it doesn't work, you don't fail—you only find one more thing that you can eliminate as a possibility.

Approaches to Successful Communication

Be Calm

Always approach your loved one in a relaxed and calm demeanor. Remember, your mood will be mirrored by your loved one. Smiles are contagious.

Be Flexible

There is no right or wrong way of completing a task. Offer praise and encouragement for the effort your loved one puts into a task. If you see your loved one becoming overwhelmed or frustrated, stop the task, and re-approach at another time.

Be Nonresistive

Don't force tasks on your loved one. Adults do not want to be told, "No!" or told what to do. The power of suggestion goes a long way, and you get more with an ounce of sugar than you do a pound of vinegar.

Be Guiding, but Not Controlling

Always use a soft, gentle approach, and remember your tone of voice. Your facial expressions must match the words you are saying.

These guidelines are effective and should be followed by you and all family members or other caregivers of your loved one. Let's look at an example of how a common approach by all caregivers can be effective in creating a positive day.

Barriers to Good Communication

Caregiver barriers and environmental barriers can negatively affect communication with your loved one. Here are some tips on how to eliminate these two barriers.

Caregiver Barriers

- Speaking too quickly. Slow down when speaking.

- Use a calm tone of voice, and be aware of your hand movements.
- Never be demanding or commanding.
- Never argue with a person with impaired cognition. You will never win the argument.
- Enter their world. Live their truth and validate.
- Do not offer long explanations when answering questions.

Environmental Barriers

- Minimize noise from air conditioners and home appliances.
- Turn off the TV if it is on in the same room where you are trying to talk.
- Be aware of outside traffic.
- Check your loved one's hearing aid battery, and make sure that it is not whistling.

- Adjust the lighting in the room. If the lighting in a room makes seeing even more difficult for someone with limited vision, they may be more focused on trying to see rather than on communicating with you.

Barriers of any type will have a negative effect on communication and could possibly lead to a behavioral issue if your loved one thinks you are yelling at them for no particular reason even though you are trying to be loud enough for them to hear you.

Let's look at an example of what we mean. One average Wednesday morning in April, you are following your normal routine of washing clothes and sheets before lunch. Your husband, Al, is sitting and watching television. It is a beautiful spring day, and you open the windows to enjoy the weather as you and Al have done for as long as you can remember on days like this. Today, there happens to be a road crew outside repaving your street. Your dogs are barking at the road crew, and the trucks in the street are running, so you turn the volume on the television up a little bit as you walk past on your way to put the last load of sheets into the washing machine. You glance at the clock and remember you have to get lunch started a little earlier today because Al has a doctor's appointment. You get the sheets in the washing machine and start making Al a turkey sandwich for lunch. You call out to him and ask what he would like to drink today with lunch. He does not answer, so you call out again, but a little louder this time.

There are four things happening at the same time: your attempt at a question, the louder-than-normal television, the road crew, and the barking dogs. This can be very overstimulating for your loved one, and they do not know where to focus, which can trigger a negative behavior. A good idea would be to shut the window for a moment to reduce the noise from the trucks and hopefully address the needs of the dogs. Then as you walk into the room smiling, turn the volume of the television down, or turn it off completely, while you explain you have a question to ask. You can then sit down at eye level with your loved one before speaking.

Validation of "Living their Truth" as a Tool to Communicating with Someone who has Alzheimer's Disease

For those we care for who have Alzheimer's, R.O.S. teaches validation as part of the communication process. Your role when working with your loved one is best expressed by author Jolene Brackey, who preaches that caregivers should take every opportunity to create moments of joy.

Many people struggle with the use of validation. There is a concern that it might appear as if you are lying to your loved one or doing them harm by not keeping them oriented to the truth. In fact, you are not lying to your loved one. You are simply meeting your loved one where they are at this moment and accepting that this is part of the illness.

As we discussed with nonverbal communication, the upside is that your actions are often mirrored by your loved one. With that knowledge—and validation—we can also address specific behavior issues.

For example, there was a man who would not eat when his wife made meals for him, and his wife began to worry about his overall health. She tried everything. She reasoned with him, she pleaded with him, and she even tried to bribe him, but nothing worked. Their daughter knew that her father was a proud man and no matter how progressed his dementia got, he was the protector, and the fixer, and had much pride with those titles. So she began coming over every day after work, and she would walk in saying, "Hi Dad," and he would respond, "Hi Babe, how are you?" That question was all she needed. She would become very dramatic and say, "Dad, let me tell you I have had a terrible day at work. I am so tired and so hungry. I did not even get lunch. My boss worked me like a dog." Immediately her father would respond, "Babe, it's not good that you cannot eat during the day. Go make yourself something to eat, and talk to me." She would proceed to make a sandwich. Cutting it into four pieces, she would put two pieces onto her plate and two pieces onto his plate. She then put a plate in front of him and a plate in front of her along with two glasses of milk, and as they started talking, her father would mimic her behavior, and they would both be eating. She would often slide another quarter of the sandwich to her father's plate without him realizing it.

Finding your loved one's motivator is important. This daily event served the purpose of getting her father to eat to maintain his health, but it also treated his soul. He could give back. He could still be the caring father, protector, and confident.

Communication and Behavior

Behaviors are a means to communicate when words are no longer effective.

Caregivers must uncover the meaning behind the behaviors and put a plan into effect to manage those needs. Be a detective.

Aggressive Behaviors

Aggressive behaviors can be defined as hitting, angry outbursts, using obscenities, yelling, verbalizing racial insults, making inappropriate sexual comments, and/or biting. Trying to communicate with or provide care to a person who is aggressive can be stressful and even frightening for caregivers.

When we meet the needs of our loved one, this type of behavior can be changed. We are the ones to ensure that our loved one still feels connected, useful, respected, and appreciated in all situations.

We have had many families and caregivers report their loved ones displaying aggressive behaviors when they are faced with a task that causes embarrassment. It has also happened when a task or activity shows their loved one is no longer independent and requires assistance. This has often occurred when trying to address the intimate issue of personal care and hygiene.

For example, there was a veteran named Bob who, prior to his Alzheimer's, lived by the U.S. Army code of hygiene, from the hair on his head, to the clothes on his body.

As his dementia got worse, he was no longer able to maintain his needs independently. Some days he would try unsuccessfully—other days he would not even make the attempt.

One of his daughters, Dana, thought focusing on his responsibility as an army man might provide him with the proper motivation.

Unfortunately, this backfired and he became belligerent and aggressive, throwing things, and cursing.

Aggressive and violent behavior can be scary, especially when it is coming from your father. We cannot forget, especially in the heat of the moment, that our loved one may look the same, they may sound the same, but because of Alzheimer's, they are not the same person. Everyone must remember that a behavior is nothing more than someone trying to tell you something with actions when they cannot say it with words.

Dana saw what was happening and remembered what she had learned about validation. She immediately validated her dad and named the behavior she was seeing.

She said, "Dad, I can see you are very angry. You wouldn't curse at me and throw things at me, or yell at me, if something was not really making you upset. Why are you so mad?"

Bob looked at her with such anger and yelled, "Because I can't do this anymore." As he spoke, his anger turned to fear and embarrassment, and with tears rolling down his face, he looked defeated, and said, "No daughter should have to bathe her father." At that moment Bob was vulnerable, and as he sat sobbing, Dana immediately put her arms around him and said, "It is my honor to assist you. We can do this together. I know you are a proud and modest man, and we will keep you covered and get this done quickly."

As she washed her father, Dana continued to talk to him as a means of distraction. She would remind him about her own memories of when she was a little girl, and he would help with bath time routines. She talked about the song that he would sing to her, and then they began to sing "Tiny Bubbles."

What started as a violent situation turned into a treasured memory for Dana and a more tolerable evening for Bob. This time things had worked out, but Dana also knew that if the anger and aggression continued, it was okay to stop and try again later.

Any caregiver may have to stop what they are trying to do with a loved one and just focus on their feelings. You may need to give them space and retry the task another time.

Possible Causes for Aggression

- Too much noise or overstimulation.
- Cluttered environment.
- Uncomfortable room temperatures.
- Basic needs not being met: hunger, thirst, needing to use the bathroom, or needing comfort.
- Pain.
- Fear, anxiety or confusion.
- Communication barriers.
- Fear or anxiety from not recognizing their surroundings.

- Caregiver's mood.
- Feeling that they are being rushed.
- Difficulty seeing activity or materials used for an activity, which may prevent them from participating.
- Lack of independence.

Interventions to Utilize to
Mitigate Aggressive Behaviors

- Validate and support their feelings.
- Reminisce with your loved one about specific details of their past.
- Remain calm, and speak in a soft tone.
- Find items that they find comfort in, e.g., a picture of the family.
- Provide consistent caregivers and schedules. Stick to your loved one's routine.
- Engage in recreational activities that match your loved one's abilities and interests, as tolerated.

- Break down instructions into one-step increments.

- Identify the triggers of the aggression. Be a detective. There is never a behavior that just occurs.

- Keep an ongoing dialogue between family members and caregivers over any noted changes in patterns or behaviors.

- Help your loved one to slow down and relax.

- Play or listen to music your loved one enjoys for its calming effects.

- Use spiritual support if this is important to your loved one.

Chapter 5

Third Pillar of Activities: Customary Routines and Preferences

Customary routines and preferences is the Third Pillar in an activities program. Activities can occur all day, every day. The question should not be, "When should I do activities?" It is not important to focus on when to do activities. The focus should be on making each and every interaction that is a part of your loved one's daily routine memorable and enjoyable.

For the purpose of developing a daily plan of care, we will be discussing two areas: Daily Customary Routine and Activity Preferences. The goal is to gain from your loved one's perspective how important certain aspects of care and activity are of interest to them as an individual.

Daily Customary Routine

Your loved one has distinct lifestyle preferences and routines. They should be preserved to the greatest extent possible. All reasonable accommodation should be made to maintain their lifestyle preferences.

Let us look at 72-year-old Sadie. Sadie's daughter, Julie, and her husband, Rick, had brought Sadie to live with their family after much discussion of, "What should we do to help Mom?" as her Alzheimer's symptoms progressed over several months. Everyone was concerned for Sadie's safety.

When Sadie moved in, there was some adjustment for everyone involved, but things smoothed out, and routines that worked for everyone were beginning to form. One of those routine items was a caregiver, Heather, coming to the house four days a week from 9:00 a.m. until 1:00 p.m. to give Julie a break.

After a few months, Sadie started doing something no one had seen before. Each morning around 10:00 a.m., Sadie would be found pacing back and forth in the hallway looking for a way out. A few times Heather found Sadie in the yard trying to get out through the locked gate. This was very distressing for everyone. No one was sure what to do, but everyone wanted to figure out the best way to protect Sadie. So Julie and Rick put locks on all of the doors in the house. This actually made the problem worse. Sadie would become very anxious, and nothing seemed to soothe her. Everyone, including Heather, the caregiver, was frustrated. This was becoming such a problem that the Heather who had built a relationship with Sadie and Julie, and was now considered part of the family, was thinking about leaving because it was becoming too much to handle.

One afternoon, Sadie and Heather were talking after lunch, and Heather starting asking Sadie about what she liked to do. Sadie said she loved to take a mid-morning daily walk in her neighborhood and then relax on her porch with a cup of tea. Heather asked Julie about this, and Julie knew that her mother had walked daily since Julie was in high school. Back then, Sadie and other ladies from the neighborhood would take a mid-morning walk after the kids were off to school. So one morning, Julie and Heather decided to take Sadie outside. "Would you like to take a walk, Sadie?" they asked as they opened the front door. Sadie hesitated, took a few steps outside with some encouragement, and then all three of them were walking. As she walked, Sadie became less anxious. After several blocks, she was smiling, talking, and laughing. Upon their return, they all sat on the porch with some tea, and Sadie seemed much more content as a result. This became a morning ritual that everyone now looked forward to.

Not accommodating your loved one's lifestyle preferences and routines can contribute to a depressed mood and increased behavioral symptoms. When a person feels like their control has been removed and that their preferences are not respected as an individual, it can be demoralizing. With Alzheimer's and other forms of dementia, caregivers must also take into consideration a person's past life and routines.

As we mentioned earlier, you typically do not know what type of day you and your loved one are going to have until it has started. That is why knowing your loved one's routines and personal history is important. Take a minute to write down some of **_your_** daily routines. It could be anything, such as:

- Your typical wake-up time.

- A morning coffee.

- Your exercise routine.

- Watching afternoon television/ talk shows.

- Working on your computer.

- Reading your social media newsfeed.

Now imagine that all of your routines abruptly and suddenly changed in one day. How would that make you feel?

Daily customary routines are something we may not think about often as they become "second nature," but they play a vital role in our daily life, stability, and quality of life.

If you were to wake up tomorrow and someone had removed all of your daily routines, there would be a variety of emotions from anger and sadness, to frustration. It's important to understand and maintain these routines as best as possible for your loved one.

Activity Preferences

Activities are a way for individuals to establish meaning in their lives. The need for enjoyable activities does not change based on your loved one's age or health needs. The only thing that

changes is the level of assistance they
may need to engage in those pursuits.

A lack of opportunity to engage in meaningful
and enjoyable activities can result in boredom,
depression, and behavioral disturbances.

Individuals vary in the activities they prefer,
reflecting unique personalities, past interests,
perceived environmental constraints, religious
and cultural background, and changing
physical and mental abilities. We as family
caregivers have a great opportunity to
empower a loved one to see that they possess
many great talents and abilities. By modifying
or adapting an activity to allow them to
engage at an independent level, you are
restoring their self-esteem and self-worth.

For example, Laura's father, Steve, was an
amazing gardener in his younger years. Steve
is 73 years old and has lived with Laura, her
two kids, and her husband, Jim, for a year. He
moved in after several small "accidents" at his

home, including a small fire when Steve left a stove burner on. Now Laura watches him dig holes in the garden. At first, she was aghast as she watched the destruction. She had always regarded her father as an amazing gardener, and she had a preconceived notion about how he should perform this activity. She could not accept her talented father operating in a primitive level. She felt she had to do something—draw his attention to the problem, show him how to do it, fix it for him, do it differently—make it turn out the way it is supposed to look. Fortunately, she stopped and observed his face as he dug the holes—he was as happy as he could be. He laughed and smiled occasionally, and focused on the task with such determination and joy that all the helplessness of the disease process—the frustration, confusion, blundering, and ugliness—disappeared. This man was back in control, enjoying a feeling of accomplishment, reveling in an activity that made sense to him. From that moment, she abandoned any notions she had had of ever seeing her father perform at his previous level of functioning. She began to regard all activity as a series of tasks that could be simplified, modified, and broken into pieces that he could find achievable.

Adaptations and modifications will be crucial for activity satisfaction and engagement. Modifications could include but aren't limited to:

- Large-print materials or a magnifying glass for reading smaller print

- Hearing aids—do they need one? Do they already have one? If your loved one has hearing aids, it is important to provide maintenance on them regularly to ensure they are working properly.

- Adequate lighting

- Hearing amplifiers

- R.O.S. Legacy System

- Card holders

- Book holders
- Large utensils
- Large-button remote controls and telephones

Identifying your loved one's needed modifications and adaptations will help them to succeed with daily life and their chosen leisure routines. Some modifications may be small, while others will be a larger undertaking. This can also be a process of trial and error, as some adaptations may work better than others. "Keep trying until the shoe fits comfortably."

Think about catching a nasty cold and how within a few days your sense of taste is gone due to the severity of the cold. You can see your favorite food; you can have a 5-star cuisine made just for you; but if you can't taste it, you're not very interested and your excitement over food diminishes.

The same concept can be understood with preferred leisure routines. You can see what you want to do; you can think about what you want to do; you can have someone there to help you; but if you don't have the proper adaptations and modifications, your interest level decreases. You have a higher risk of agitation, self-isolation, depression, and frustration.

Chapter 6

Fourth Pillar of Activities: Planning and Executing Activities

Planning and executing activities is the Fourth Pillar in engaging a loved one in an activity. With the knowledge of your loved one's history, functional level, effective communication techniques to use, and their daily routine, we now look at planning activities in which they can be successful.

The Lesson Plan

The Lesson Plan template is a guideline for an activity. Our loved one's abilities and responses may differ from day to day or even hour to hour. This will dictate how you modify an activity to meet their individual needs and abilities.

Here is an example. Sixty-four-year-old Amy enjoyed art activities. She especially loved to paint. She had volunteered as an art teacher at a local preschool for years. Her husband, Joe, who was Amy's primary caregiver, knew this, but was not sure how to get Amy to do anything with art because he had never painted or helped children with art projects. That had always been Amy's specialty. Joe would get tired of Amy always sitting and watching TV, but every time he asked, "Would you like to paint a picture?" she said, "No." One afternoon, at a support group meeting, he heard a discussion about activity lesson plans and how they included step-by-step instructions on engaging someone in an activity they might enjoy. Joe found a lesson plan for a painting activity and decided to give it a try. He gathered all of the materials called for in the lesson plan and laid them out on a table. He brought Amy to the table and asked for her help to paint a picture. Joe had prepared everything, and all of the supplies were there to get started—some tempera paint poured into cups of assorted colors, a brush, and a piece of canvas placed on an easel. Joe knew Amy loved daisies, so he told her he wanted to create a painting of a vase full of daises, but was not sure how to get started. He placed the brush in Amy's hand, pointed toward one of the cups of paint, and asked if she would get him started. Amy dipped the brush into the paint and went to town on the canvas. She worked until the canvas was completely covered in a myriad of colors. Amy seemed pretty satisfied once she was "done."

Joe took the brush to the sink to wash it out and upon his return was horrified to see Amy taking a sip from the orange paint. "Thank goodness that tempera paint is nontoxic," he thought. "Lesson learned." He now knew that if they were to do a similar art activity again, he would have to provide extra supervision with regard to the paint. This tidbit of information was then written into the evaluation portion of the lesson plan so that it was a written reminder for him and any others caregivers.

The Lesson Plan is an ever-changing document. It is meant to be written on to note any changes needed so the next person working with your loved one can follow your modifications in hopes of recreating a positive experience.

Items in the Lesson Plan

Date

Document the date the activity is used.

Activity Name

You can rename the activity if you or your loved one prefers.

Objective of Activity

Our goal is to provide meaningful activities. People have a need to be productive, and they want to engage in something with a purpose. List the objectives of the activity.

Materials

The list of suggested materials to use with this activity.

Prerequisite Skills

The skills your loved one needs to participate in this activity.

Activity Outline

Step-by-step instructions to complete this activity.

Evaluation

When you or a family member are conducting an activity with your loved one, documenting results and responses is critical to improve activity programs for your loved one. Items to document:

- Verbal cues, physical assistance or modifications you make to activity.

- Your loved one's response to this activity.

- Did your loved one enjoy this activity or not?

- Was the activity successful at distracting or eliminating a negative behavior?

A blank template is included on the next page to give you an example of what a Lesson Plan looks like.

Lesson Plan Blank Example

Date	Activity Name

Objective of Activity

Materials

Prerequisite Skills

Activity Outline

Evaluation

Lesson Plan Example

Date	Activity Name
9/21/15	**Mind Challenge**

Objective of Activity *(1) Promotion of independent thinking, (2) Brain exercise, (3) Opportunity for success*

Materials *(1) 5x7 note cards, (2) 1 marker or Sharpie, (3) Pencil or pen for loved one*

Prerequisite Skills *(1) Listening skills, (2) Hand movement, (3) Motor skills*

Activity Outline *(1) On the top of each note card write a word with a black marker (any word, preferably a long word), (2) Provide loved one with the note card and a pencil or pen, (3) Direct loved one to make smaller words out of the letters from the word on the note card, (4) This is a great activity to do together or independently.*

Evaluation *Mr. Smith enjoyed doing this activity today. He does display a short attention span during nonphysical programs. It's beneficial to sit with him and participate in this activity together—he responds well to having assistance.*

Lesson Plan Example

Date	Activity Name
9/22/15	**Birdhouses**

Objective of Activity *(1) Promote visual and tactile stimulation, (2) Male-oriented activity, (3) Provide an opportunity for reminiscing*

Materials *(1) Unfinished wooden birdhouse, (2) Sandpaper, (3) Paint, (4) Paintbrush, (5) Cup of water—for rinsing the brush, (6) Newspaper or plastic tablecloth*

Prerequisite Skills *(1) Hand coordination, (2) Hand/Eye coordination*

Activity Outline *(1) Cover your activity area surface with a newspaper or plastic tablecloth, (2) Sand the birdhouse until smooth, (3) Use the paint color of preference to paint the birdhouse.*

Evaluation *Mr. Smith got frustrated and didn't like the feel of the sandpaper. I skipped this step today and allowed him to paint the birdhouse without the sanding. He enjoyed the painting, and his mood improved once the sandpaper was gone. Since he was so engaged in painting the house, painting activities would be good for the future without the birdhouse.*

Chapter 7

Leisure Activity
Categories, Types, Topics, and Tips

Activity Categories

Activities are generally broken down into three different categories: Maintenance Activities, Supportive Activities, and Empowering Activities.

Maintenance Activities

Maintenance activities are traditional activities that help your loved one maintain physical, cognitive, social, spiritual, and emotional health. Examples include:

- Using manipulative games, such as those in the R.O.S. Legacy System

- Craft and art activities

- Attending church services

- Working trivia and crossword puzzles like the *How Much Do You Know About* puzzles

- Taking a walk

- Tai chi

Maintenance activities are so important. As caregivers, we must continue to try even if we have to modify an activity our loved one had done their whole life. Let us consider Carol who was an avid church goer who had been actively involved in the choir. She grew up with all of the old church hymns and knew many of them by heart. Although her Alzheimer's has progressed to the point where she no longer has the focus of attention to sit through a complete worship service and sermon, she can stay for the musical worship part of the service and sing freely without using a hymnal book. It is amazing to see how alive Carol becomes through the spirit of music.

Supportive Activities

Supportive activities are for those that have a lower tolerance for traditional activities. These types of activities provide a comfortable environment while providing stimulation or solace. Examples include:

- Listening to and singing music
- Hand massages
- Relaxation activities, such as aromatherapy, meditation, and bird-watching

Liza grew up on a farm and especially loved her herb garden. She had been an expert at using different herbs for cooking and making different types of teas. Liza was no longer able to cook or move around a garden, but her caregiver knew that she enjoyed the warmth of the sun on her face and gardening, so she brought Liza outside on nice days. She would also bring different types of herbs for her to smell, touch, and taste as part of a pre-lunch activity. The caregiver knew basil was Liza's favorite so there was always plenty of basil as part of the activity, which led to a conversation about cooking and different recipes for meals that included basil.

Empowering Activities

Empowering activities help your loved one attain self-respect by receiving opportunities for self-expression and responsibility. Examples include:

- Cooking
- Making memory boxes
- Folding laundry

Grace, a mother of four and grandmother of ten, liked to do her own laundry. She would sort the dark clothes from the light clothes, pick out her own detergent, and measure the detergent herself with some simple cues. Once her laundry was washed, sorted, and folded, she would place the clean clothes neatly in her cabinet. Each and every time she had visitors, Grace would open the cabinet drawers to proudly show them the work that she did.

Activity Types

Once you have chosen an activity from a category that will suit your loved one's need, you must choose an activity type that will interest them. There are several types of activities to choose from. Below are some examples:

Art Activities

- Coloring
- Painting
- Dancing
- Clay Sculpting
- Drawing

Craft Activities

- Jewelry making
- Knitting

- Scrapbooking
- Birdhouses
- Woodworking
- Home décor
- Decoupage
- Quilting
- Needleworking
- Wreath making
- Models (cars/planes)

Verbal Activities

- Conversation
- Trivia
- Reminiscing

Entertainment Activities

- Board games
- Card games
- Video games
- Crossword puzzles
- Movies
- Computer Apps

Listening Activities

- Music
- Storytelling
- Books on tape
- Listening to the radio

Visual Activities

- Watching a movie
- Watching a performance

Writing Activities

- Writing a story or poem
- Writing a letter
- Life stories

Active Activities

- Dancing
- Folding laundry
- Road trips
- Exercise
- Ball games
- Tai chi
- Sittercise

Activity Topics

Once you know what category of activity you want to engage your loved one from, here are some suggestions for topics the activity can be based on:

Colors

- Colors of their favorite sports team
- Colors of their wedding
- Colors of flowers or cars

Music

- Favorite music
- Music from when they were younger and dating
- Patriotic songs
- Holiday songs
- Favorite artists from the age they think they are, e.g., if they believe they are 25 years old, use popular singers or songs of that era.

Military Service

- War stories—if this is a topic they are comfortable discussing and recounting events
- World events of their time
- Their personal experiences of either military service or what it was like in the States

Holidays

- Specific holidays that coincide with their culture or religion
- Favorite holidays
- Family holiday traditions
- Most memorable holiday memory

Cooking

- Home cooking
- Comfort food
- Favorite recipes from their mother/grandmother

- Favorite food associated with events, holidays, family gatherings
- Making a cookbook with loved one to pass on to the family

Sports

- Professional sports teams they liked
- Their involvement in sports
- Big sporting events from their era

School Days

- Where they went to school
- Favorite school classes or teachers
- Memories of their children's school events

Old Cars

- Their family's first car
- Their first car
- Prices of cars now and then
- Dream cars

Places

- Where they were born
- Where they grew up
- Places they have been
- Vacations they took

Activity Tips for Individuals with Mild to Moderate Alzheimer's Disease

Many loved ones have cognitive deficits that are significant enough to impact their day as well as their awareness of their surroundings. By providing activities that reinforce their past, we increase and improve their social skills which can improve their general interactions with others.

Validating Activities

Validating activities validate the memories and feelings of individuals who are much disoriented. They focus on your loved one's perception of what happened in the past.

Validating is stepping into the reality that your loved one is in. Avoid confrontation, and validate their feelings and statements.

Reminiscing Activities

Reminiscing activities are designed to help your loved one identify the important contributions he or she has made throughout their lifetime. It is an important part of human development to see oneself as a contributing member of society.

A great reminiscing activity to do with your loved one is a memory box. Memory boxes can hold a variety of memorabilia from your loved one's personal life, e.g., photos, medals, clothing articles, newspaper clips, and jewelry. You can also make your own topic-specific memory boxes based on topics that matter to your loved one, such as sports, back to school, cooking, history, or fashion.

Resocializing Activities

Once your loved one can successfully participate in reminiscing and validating activities, it is time to encourage them, through resocializing activities, to build on those social skills, and begin to expand their connections to the community in which they live. This can be as simple as with a neighbor, in church, or within their community.

Chapter 8

Activities of Daily Living
Tips and Suggestions

Unlike leisure activities, the activities of daily living covered in this book are necessary activities that are a part of everyday life. The following pages contain tips and suggestions for you to use with your loved one.

Bathing

Bathing can be a relaxing, enjoyable experience—or a time of confrontation and anger. Use a calm approach. Your loved one's "usual" routine is very important.

Safety

- Water temperature should range from 110–115 degrees Fahrenheit maximum to prevent burning or skin injury.

- The floor of the tub needs to be slip proof. Use a rubber mat that does not slide, or use permanent nonslip decals.

- Place a nonskid rug on the floor outside the tub to prevent slipping.

- Install grab bars. Always make sure the grab bars are properly and securely installed into the wall studs.

- Do not use bath oils.

Never leave your loved one unattended in the bathroom.

Bathing—Know Your Loved One

- Is your loved one accustomed to a bath or shower?

- Can they get into a bath or shower without assistance?

- Who is your loved one the most comfortable with when needing care? Is it a female or a male—or a specific caregiver?

***Note:** Sex and age of the caregiver can be a significant issue. For example, a 90-year-old female might be horrified if a 20-year-old male family member came into the bathroom to assist with care. She may fear for her safety or be embarrassed depending on her level of dementia.

Bathing—Communicating and Motivating

- Don't ask if they want to bathe. Simply say in an easy, friendly voice, "Bath time."

- Use short, simple sentences.

- Look directly at your loved one.

- Be mindful of the little details— preparation and execution.

- Always smile, talk calmly and gently.

- Do not argue, or try to explain "why."

- If your loved one becomes angry or combative about bathing, **_STOP_** and try another time.

Bathing—Customary Routines and Preferences

- What time of day does the loved one normally bathe?

- Does your loved one wash their hair or body first?

Bathing—Planning and Executing

- Consider the process that works for the caregiver and loved one when it is time to bathe.

For example, your loved one needs assistance undressing and getting into the tub. They always remove their shirt first, followed by their pants, socks, and underwear. The tub has a built-in seat that is covered with ceramic tile. Your loved one needs a towel laid on the tile prior to sitting down because the tile is cold against their skin. Once seated, your loved one also likes a towel draped over their shoulders so they feel less exposed with you assisting them while they bathe.

- Have all care items and tools ready prior to starting the bath process.
- Have a shower chair if necessary.
- Have a handheld hose for showering and bathing.
- Have a long-handled sponge or scrubbing brush if they would like to scrub themselves.
- Have sponges with soap inside or a soft soap applicator instead of bar soap. Bar soap can easily slip out of your loved one's hand.
- One step at a time, follow their normal routine. Wash hair first, and then wash body, or soak for 10 minutes before washing? When they finish one step, go to the next.
- Remember to **_STOP_** and try another time if your loved one becomes angry or combative.
- Have towel and clothing prepared for when the bath is finished.

- Use a terry cloth robe instead of a towel to dry off.

Other Bathroom & Grooming Activities

Brushing Teeth

- Give them step-by-step directions. This may not be as simple as you think. Take a moment and think of all of the steps necessary to brush your teeth, from walking into the bathroom, to finding the toothpaste in the drawer and removing the cap, to rinsing their mouth once they have finished brushing. Depending on your loved one's level of Alzheimer's, it might be easier to show them.

- For family members at home, brush your teeth at the same time.

- Use positive reinforcement and compliment your loved one on the good job they are doing.

- Help your loved one to clean their dentures as needed.

Shaving

- Encourage a male to shave.
- Use an electric razor for safety.
- If they need assistance, please provide it.
- Give positive feedback, and do not verbally correct.

For example, if your loved one only managed to shave half of his face, do not criticize and tell him he "did it wrong." Instead, ask if he would like some help.

Makeup

- If your loved one had been accustomed to wearing makeup prior to the onset of Alzheimer's, there is no reason for this to stop. If she shows interest or desire to wear makeup, encourage her to do so, and offer assistance to apply if needed.

Hair

- Try to maintain hairstyle and care as your loved one did.

- Explain each step simply beforehand to reduce any anxiety.

- When washing hair, use nonstinging shampoo.

- Use warm water for washing and rinsing. Tell your loved one before you rinse their hair.

Nails

- Keep nails clean and trimmed. Be gentle while trimming your loved one's nails. Be mindful of how you pull and where you place their fingers and arms.

- If your loved one had a normal/weekly schedule for nail care prior to the onset of Alzheimer's or other health issues, please try to maintain that schedule.

- Offer to polish your loved one's nails.

- When polishing, engage your loved one in conversation.

Toileting or Using the Bathroom

- Mark the bathroom door so it can be identified.

- Learn your loved one's individual habits and routines for using the toilet. This may not be something that you knew before and is part of the changing roles.

- Toilet routinely on rising, before and after meals, and at bedtime, at a minimum.

- If your loved one is having trouble communicating, please watch for agitation, pulling at their clothes, or walking/pacing restlessly. This may be an indication that they need to go to the bathroom.

- Assist with clothing as needed, and be positive and pleasant while assisting.

- Provide verbal cues and instructions as needed, while being guiding, but not controlling as you do.

Clothing

Clothing—Know Your Loved One

- Daily clothing choices should remain as they had been before the onset of Alzheimer's and based on your loved one's available wardrobe during the initial stages of the disease.

- As their Alzheimer's progresses, changes will have to be made. Clothes need to be comfortable and easy to remove, especially to go to bathroom.

Clothing—Routines and Preferences

- Have a friendly discussion each evening about the next day's schedule and what your loved one may want to wear.

- Remember that as their Alzheimer's progresses, changes will have to be made. You may have to limit the choice of clothing, and leave only two outfit options in their room at a time.

- If your loved one wants to wear the same thing every day, and if you can afford it, buy three or four sets of the same clothing.

- Try to maintain your loved one's preferred dressing routine by laying the clothes out in order of what your loved one prefers to put on first.

Clothing—Planning and Executing

- Choose clothes that are loose fitting and have elastic waistbands.

- Choose wraparound clothing instead of the pullover type.

- You may consider clothing that opens and closes in the front, not the back, for your loved one. This prevents your loved one from having to reach behind their body and allows the feeling of independence from dressing oneself.

- When purchasing new clothes, look for clothing with large, flat buttons; Velcro closures, or zippers.

- If possible, attach a zipper pull to the end of the zipper to make it easier to zip pants or jackets.

- Choose slip-on shoes, and purchase elastic shoelaces that allow shoes to slip on and off without untying the shoelaces.

Dressing

Dressing—Know Your Loved One

Initially, your loved one may just need verbal cues and instructions on dressing. As their Alzheimer's progresses, you will have to take a more active role. Please remember to allow your loved one to dress independently as long as possible to foster an ongoing sense of dignity and independence. You will have to be the judge of when all caregivers need to begin assisting in the dressing process.

Similar to bathing, you need to identify who your loved one is the most comfortable with when needing care. Is it a female or a male— or a specific caregiver?

Sex and age of the caregiver can be a significant issue.

Dressing—Communicating and Motivating

- Use short, simple sentences.

- Provide verbal cues and instructions as needed.

- Ask if your loved one would like to go to the toilet before getting dressed.

- If your loved one is confused, give instructions in very short steps, such as, "Now put your arm through the sleeve." It may help to use actions to demonstrate these instructions.

- Give praise as justified as each step is accomplished.

- Always smile, talk calmly and gently.

- Do not argue, or try to explain "why."

- Be guiding, not controlling.

Dressing—Routines and Preferences

- Does your loved one get dressed first thing in the morning—before breakfast or after breakfast?

- Does your loved one change into pajamas right before bed or after dinner?

- Try to maintain your loved one's preferred routine. For example, they may like to put on all of their underwear before putting on anything else.

Dressing—Planning and Executing

- Think about privacy—make sure that blinds or curtains are closed and that no one will walk in and disturb your loved one while they are dressing.

- Make sure the room is warm enough to get dressed in.

- Before handing your loved one their clothes, make sure that items are not inside out and that buttons, zips, and fasteners are all undone.

- Hand your loved one a single item at a time.

- To assist with balance, let your loved one get dressed while sitting in a chair that has armrests.

If mistakes are made—for example, something is put on the wrong way—be tactful, or find a way for you both to laugh about it.

*Note: It can be helpful if your loved one wears several layers of thin clothing rather than one thick layer. With layers, your loved one can remove a layer if they feel too warm.

Remember that your loved one may get to a point where they are no longer able to tell you if they are too hot or cold, so keep an eye out for signs of discomfort.

Meals

General Information

- Limit distractions. Serve meals in quiet surroundings, away from the television and other activities.

- Your loved one might not be able to tell if something is too hot to eat or drink. Always test the temperature of foods and beverages before serving.

- Keep long-standing personal preferences in mind when preparing food. **_However_**, be aware that your loved one may suddenly develop new food preferences or reject foods that were liked in the past.

- Give your loved one plenty of time to eat. It may take an hour or longer to finish a snack or meal.

- Make meals an enjoyable social event so everyone looks forward to the experience.

Eating

Eating—Know Your Loved One

- Can your loved one feed themselves?

- Does your loved one have a visual impairment that may affect their ability to see their meal or drink?

  *Note: Older individuals tend to perceive bright, deep colors as lighter. They are able to see yellow, orange, and red more easily than darker colors. Due to normal changes in our eyesight as we age, eating and dining may offer additional challenges.

Meals—Communicating and Motivating

- Use short, simple sentences.

- Provide verbal cues and instructions as needed.

- Give your loved one your full attention.

- Always smile, talk calmly and gently.

- Do not argue, or try to explain "why."

Meals—Routines and Preferences

- No matter what time of day breakfast, lunch, and dinner are served, be consistent every day.
- Offer snacks throughout the day.
- Do they eat their meals at the kitchen table?
- It may take an hour or longer to finish a snack or meal so factor that into the overall schedule of the day.

Meals—Planning and Executing

Eating a meal can be a challenge for your loved one with Alzheimer's. There are several areas that need to be taken into account, such as visual impairment, physical ailment, changes in preferences, and dietary restrictions. Here are some simple techniques that can help reduce mealtime problems:

Meal Preparation for Mild Alzheimer's

- If your loved one wants to assist in making a meal:

123

- Make sure your cabinets are organized with each item labeled with large easy-to-see labels.
- Use simple written or verbal step-by-step instructions.
- You or another caregiver must perform tasks using sharp objects, such as knives, and assume operation of the stove or oven.
- When using a stove top, use the back burners, and turn the pot handles inward toward the back of the stove to avoid any potential grabbing of the pots or pans.

- If you are not there to supervise because you have to go to work:

  - Avoid planning meals that require use of the stove. Your loved one may not remember to turn off the stove and may not be able to distinguish between a pot that is hot or cold.

- Lay out the ingredients of a meal on the counter or in the refrigerator in labeled containers in the order that your loved one will use them—similar to laying out their clothes at night.

- Transfer bulk items, including milk, from a larger container to a smaller container that is easier to lift and pour.

Meal Preparation for Higher Level Alzheimer's

- Try to have all meals eaten at a kitchen or dining table, or a chair with a serving tray.

- Avoid meals in bed, if possible—let the bed be for sleeping.

Appropriate Lighting and Eyesight

- Reduce glare by having your loved one sit with the sunlight behind them when eating.

- Use lighting which illuminates the entire dining space and makes objects visible, as well as reducing shadows or reflections.

- Adjust lighting above the table to help see as much detail as possible.

- Remember that older individuals tend to perceive bright, deep colors as lighter. They are able to see yellow, orange, and red more easily than darker colors.

Setting the Table and Serving

- Set each place setting in the same way for every meal. Set it the way your loved one used to, and offer them the opportunity to assist in setting the table.

- Decide how to set the rest of the table— main dish, side dishes, seasonings, and condiments. Do it the same way each day.

- When pouring a light-colored drink, such as milk, use a dark glass.

- When pouring a dark-colored drink, such as cola, use a white glass.

- Avoid clear glasses. They can disappear from view.

- Use white dishes when eating dark-colored food, and use dark dishes when eating light-colored food.

- To make dishes easier to find on the table, use a tablecloth or placemats that are the opposite color of the dishes.

- Fiesta ware colors (yellow/tangerine) contrast with most foods so they can be easily seen and will enhance visual perception.

- There should be a clear visual distinction between the table, the dishes, and the food.

- Use solid colors with no distracting patterns.

Chapter 9

Home Preparation

The home is your loved one's castle. This is something they are familiar with and feel comfortable in. Keeping the home a haven can become difficult as your loved one moves into the final stages of the disease process. Whether you live in a house, an apartment, or an independent living facility, you and your loved one need to feel comfortable, capable, and safe. This is a foundational piece of preparation to have your loved one engage in an activity. The following are general tips that caregivers and family members can use to prepare the home as your loved one's Alzheimer's progresses.

General Organization and Environment

When organizing your loved one's environment, be sure to do it **with** them. What works for you, may not work for your loved one.

- Assign everything to a place in the home. Always put items back in their place after using them in order to avoid clutter.

- Remove objects left on the floor, such as shoes, bags, and boxes. They should be placed in their designated areas of the home. If left out, they can be a tripping hazard.

- Use extension cords sparingly, and always secure them out of the places where people walk. Bundle all the cords, and secure them to the wall instead of the floor.

- Organize like objects in the same area whenever possible so that they are easily located.

- Remove and avoid clutter on desks, tables, and countertops, and in cabinets and closets. This makes it easier to locate and reach specific items.

- Avoid the use of throw rugs. They can be a tripping hazard when moving from room to room for an activity. If you must use them, opt for slide-resistant rugs that can be taped or tacked down.

- Install handrails where possible for easier independent movement from one room to the next.

- Leave doors fully opened or closed. Make sure the doors open easily and smoothly and that doorknobs are securely fastened to the door.

- Identify and address flooring issues. Check every floor, walkway, threshold, and entry. Remove or fix loose floorboards, uneven tiles, loose nails, or carpeting that has bunched up over time.

Furniture

- Make sure there is enough room to move around. If your loved one uses a wheelchair, and if possible, place furniture pieces 5½ feet from each other so your loved one can move comfortably around the room.

- Use chairs with straight backs, armrests, and firm seats. Where possible, add firm cushions to existing pieces to add height. This will make it easier for your loved one to sit down and get up.

Lighting

Depending on your loved one's eye condition, Alzheimer's symptoms or individual preference, the need for additional or less lighting could be key in their safety and ability to perform tasks independently.

- Fluorescent lighting can contribute to an increase in glare. Try different types of bulbs to see which is most comfortable for your loved one.

- Keep all rooms evenly lit and lighting level consistent throughout the house so shadows and dangerous bright spots are eliminated.

- Make sure light switches, pull cords, and lamps are easily accessible for your loved one in case they are in a wheelchair.

- If possible, purchase touch lamps or those that can be turned on or off by sound.

- Depending on the individual, additional task lighting may be necessary in certain areas of the home.

Glare

Glare can be caused by sunlight or light from a lamp. Glare can make it difficult for an individual with low vision to see when the glare hits shiny surfaces, including glossy paint on walls. Sunglasses can be beneficial both indoors and outside for someone who is light sensitive.

- Enable sunlight to fill the room with light without producing glare. Adjust sunlight coming from windows by using mini blinds and altering their position throughout the day. If mini blinds are not available, use sheer curtains.

- Be aware when placing mirrors in a room. Mirrors placed across from larger windows can significantly increase the amount of light in a room, but they can also be the source of a significant amount of glare.

- Cover bare lightbulbs of all types with shades.

- Position chairs and tables so that when your loved one is sitting on a chair or at a table, they are not having to look directly at the light coming from the window.

- Cover or remove shiny/reflective surfaces, such as floors and tabletops.

Color Contrasts

Using contrast is a key strategy if your loved one has a visual impairment. The more contrast, the easier it is to find and use objects or activity items around the house.

- Put light-colored objects against a dark background.

- Avoid upholstery with patterns for seated activities. Stripes, plaids, and checks can be visually confusing.

- Opt for solid-colored tables and countertops in a neutral tone. Countertops with busy patterns can make it difficult to locate items and can be more difficult to keep clean.

- In a room with mostly dark tones, place light-colored pillows or chairs in strategic places to help your loved one find things and get around easily.

Chapter 10

Put Your Mask on First

There will be many challenges to you personally in this caregiving journey that can and will wear you down. As a caregiver, first and foremost, you must take care of yourself in order to be able to assist your loved one. That might be easier said than done, but please make every effort to do so. The following are some general tips for you, the family caregiver:

About You

- Put yourself first (this is not being selfish) —if you are not in good physical or mental health you cannot help anyone.
- Arrange some time for yourself.
- Keep a strong support system.
- Do not be afraid to ask for help.
- Keep contact with friends.
- Define priorities; do not try to be all things to all people.

Stress

- Recognize your own stress and take steps to minimize. Stress can be exhibited in multiple ways:
  - Anger
  - Helplessness
  - Embarrassment
  - Grief
  - Depression
  - Isolation
  - Physical illness

Burnout

Burnout for caregivers results from physical and emotional exhaustion.

It is important to realize a family member, spouse, or hired caregiver experiences the same emotions as staff in health care facilities, but may not have the needed support system. Suggestions to avoid burnout:

- Know what makes you angry or impatient. Make a list.

- Look for the reason behind behavior.
- Use relaxation techniques, e.g., deep breathing, imagery, and music.
- Ask for help, and accept help when it is offered!

Caregiving is a challenging road with constant twists and turns, from the change in your role/relationship with your loved one, to dealing with the strains of a 24/7 job of caring for that loved one. As much as you may feel like you are alone, please know that you are not. Millions of family caregivers are dealing with the same issues that you are. Do not be embarrassed to share details about what you are experiencing, and do not be afraid to ask for help. There are individuals, organizations, and support groups throughout the country that are available to you. There is also R.O.S. —we were built on the simple mission of our founder's need to help his mother and father during a 25-year battle with Parkinson's and dementia. We understand what you are going through, and we are here to help.

Personal History Form

This is _____ 's Personal History

Name:_____

Maiden Name:_____

Date of Birth:_____

Preferred Name: _____

Name and relationship of people completing this history:

_____

_____

_____

What age do you think the person thinks they are?

_____

Do they ask for their spouse but do not recognize them?

_____

Do they look for their children but do not recognize them?

_____

Do they look for their mom? _____

Do they perceive themselves as younger? Please describe.

_____

_____

Describe the "home" they remember. _____

_____

_____

_____

Describe the person's personality prior to the onset of
Alzheimer's disease. _____

_____

_____

What makes the person feel valued? Talents, occupation,
accomplishments, family, etc. _____

_____

_____

What are some favorite items the person must always
have in sight or close by? _____

_____

_____

What is their exact morning daily routine? _____

_____

_____

_____

_____

What is their exact evening routine?

_____

_____

_____

_____

What type of clothing does this person prefer? Do they like to choose their own clothes for the day, or do they prefer to have their clothes laid out for them?

_____

_____

_____

_____

What is their favorite beverage?

_____

What is their favorite food?

_____

What will get them motivated? (Church, friends coming over, going out, etc.)?

_____

_____

_____

_____

List significant interests in their life, such as hobbies, recreational activities, job related skills/experiences, military experience, etc.

   - Age 8 to 20:

   _____

   _____

   _____

   - Age 20 to 40:

   _____

   _____

   _____

What is their religious background? (Affiliation, prayer time, symbols, traditions, church/synagogue name, etc.) Did they lead any services or sing in the choir?)

   _____

   _____

   _____

What type of music do they enjoy listening to, playing, or singing? Do they have any musical talents?

   _____

   _____

   _____

What is their favorite TV program? Movie?

_____

_____

_____

Did they enjoy reading? Which authors, topics, or genres do they prefer? Would they listen to audiobooks or books on tape?

_____

_____

_____

_____

Can they tell the difference between someone on TV and a real person?

_____

_____

Marital status—If married more than once, provide specifics. Include names of spouses, dates of marriage, and other relevant information.

_____

_____

_____

_____

_____

List distinct characteristics about their spouse(s), such as occupations, personality traits, or daily routine.

_____

_____

_____

_____

_____

Do they have children? Be sure to include children both living and deceased. Include names, birth dates, and any other relevant information.

_____

_____

_____

_____

_____

Who do they ask for the most? What is their relationship with this person(s)? Describe how that person typically spends their day.

_____

_____

_____

_____

_____

What causes your loved one stress?

_____

_____

_____

_____

What calms them down when they are stressed or agitated?

_____

_____

_____

_____

Other information that would help bring joy to your loved one.

_____

_____

_____

_____

_____

_____

_____

_____

_____

_____

About the Authors

Scott Silknitter

Scott Silknitter is the founder of R.O.S. Therapy Systems. He designed and created the R.O.S. Play Therapy™ System, the *How Much Do You Know About* Series of themed activity books, and the R.O.S. *BIG Book*. Starting with a simple backyard project to help his mother and father, Scott has dedicated his life to improving the quality of life for all seniors through meaningful education, entertainment, and activities.

Cindy Bradshaw, MS, ACC

Cindy Bradshaw is the Executive Director of the National Certification Council for Activity Professionals (NCCAP). She is an Activity Consultant and educator and a leader in the field of activities. Cindy co-developed and teaches the Modular Education Program for Activity Professionals (MEPAP 2nd Edition) and the Home Care Certification (HCC) curriculum. With over 30 years of experience in Geriatrics, Cindy has lobbied state and federal governments to set quality of life standards for senior residents and clients of all long-term care settings.

Alisa Tagg, BA, ACC/EDU, AC-BC, CDP

Alisa Tagg currently serves as the President of the National Association of Activity Professionals (NAAP). She is a Certified Activity Consultant with a specialization in Education and a Certified Dementia

Practitioner. With over 20 years of industry experience, Alisa is an authorized certification instructor for the Modular Education Program for Activity Professionals. Alisa speaks on local, state, and national levels on various topics relating to health care, the activity profession, and the social model of care.

Dawn Worsley, ADC/MC/EDU, CDP

Dawn Worsley currently serves as the President of the National Certification Council for Activity Professionals. She is a Certified Activity Director with a specialization in Education and Memory Care, a Certified Eden Alternative Associate, a Certified Dementia Care Practitioner, and an Alzheimer's Dementia Care Trainer. With over 20 years of experience, Ms. Worsley is an authorized certification instructor with the National Council of Certified Dementia Practitioners (NCCDP) and a Modular Education Program for Activity Professionals course instructor.

Vanessa Emm, BA, ACC/EDU, AC-BC, CDP

Vanessa Emm currently serves as the Operations Trustee for the National Association of Activity Professionals. She is a Certified Activity Consultant/Instructor/Educator through NCCAP, a Consultant through the National Association of Activity Professionals Credentialing Center (NAAPCC), and a Certified Dementia Practitioner through the NCCDP. With over 12 years of experience in long-term care,

Vanessa currently works as an Activity Consultant. She has presented at national conferences, state conferences, and workshops.

Linda Redhead, MS, ACC/EDU

Linda Redhead is a Board Member of the National Certification Council for Activity Professionals Special Projects. She is a certified Activity Professional and a Certified Activity Consultant with a specialization in education. With over 22 years of activity experience in long-term care, Linda is a Modular Education Program for Activity Professionals course instructor and was the 2013 MEPAP instructor of the year.

Robert D. Brennan, RN, NHA, MS, CDP

Robert Brennan was responsible for the development of an Assisted Living Federation of America (ALFA) "Best of the Best" award-winning program for care of individuals with dementia using Montessori-Based Dementia Programming (MBDP). He is a Registered Nurse and Nursing Home Administrator with over 35 years of experience in long-term care. He is a Certified Dementia Practitioner and is Credentialed in MBDP. He currently provides education on dementia and long-term regulatory topics.

References

1. *The Handbook of Theories on Aging* (Bengtson et al., 2009)
2. *Activity Keeps Me Going & Going, Volume 1*, (Peckham et al., 2011)
3. *Essentials for the Activity Professional in Long-Term Care* (Lanza, 1997)
4. *Abnormal Psychology*, Butcher
5. www.dhspecialservices. com
6. National Certification Council for Dementia Practitioners, www.NCCDP.org
7. "Managing Difficult Dementia Behaviors: An A-B-C Approach" By Carrie Steckl
8. Iowa Geriatric Education Center website, Marianne Smith, PhD, ARNP, BC Assistant Professor University of Iowa College of Nursing
9. *Excerpts taken from "Behavior...Whose Problem is it?" Hommel, 2012
10. *Merriam-Webster's Dictionary*
11. "The Latent Kin Matrix" (Riley, 1983)
12. *Care Planning Cookbook* (Nolta et al. 2007)
13. "Long-Term Care" (Blasko et al. 2011)
14. "Success-Oriented Programs for the Dementia Client" (Worsley et al 2005)
15. Heerema, Esther. "Eight Reasons Why Meaningful Activities Are Important for People with Dementia." www.about.com
16. *Validation: The Feil Method* (Feil, 1992)
17. *Activities 101 for the Family Caregiver* (Appler-Worsley, Bradshaw, Silknitter)
18. American Foundation for the Blind
19. www.aging.com
20. www.WebMD.com
21. www.nia.nih.gov
22. www.caregiver.org

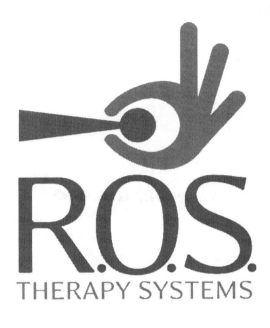

For additional assistance, please contact us at:
www.ROSTherapySystems.com
888-352-9788

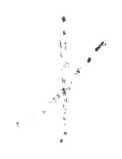

Made in the USA
Charleston, SC
29 December 2015